SICK? STAY HOME!

AND WAYS TO STAY WELL

KOLYA LYNNE SMITH

Contents

ABOUT THE AUTHOR

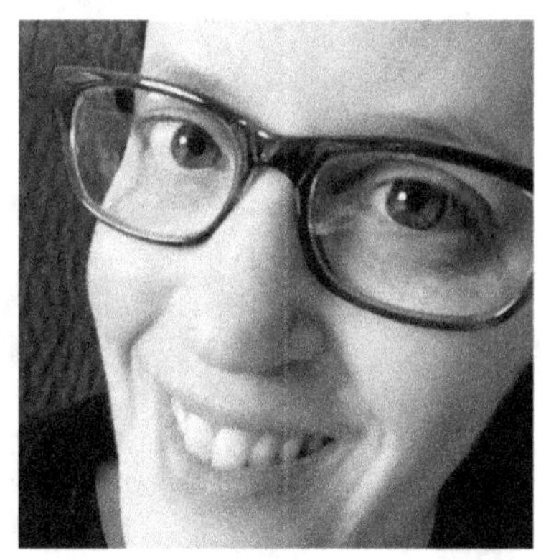

Kolya Lynne Smith lives in Boston, Massachusetts. In 2003, she was diagnosed with multiple sclerosis. A year prior, she was also diagnosed with Arnold Chiari malformation. For almost 5 years, she was the director of Ehrick Garion's Act, a medical advocacy nonprofit organization, which advocated for people who have this neurological condition. She was the first person to speak at a sociological conference on the topic. The medical field has always been a part of her life. Her high school degree was in medical secretary. Her college degree was in sociology with an applied focus in medical sociology. She has worked at several hospitals and health facilities as a switchboard operator or secretary. Her love for research has taught her a lot about illness and how to stay well. After getting sick repeatedly, she started to write this book, which is an outgrowth of her passion for medical advocacy.

INTRODUCTION

Note: This introduction was written pre-pandemic (2018).

I'm on the train and all I hear is a symphony of coughs, sneezes, and sniffles. It's like an incubator for germs. I can't wait until it's my stop to get off! The young woman across from me is too busy with her cell phone to stop and cover her cough. She would rather text someone. Meanwhile, a young man is coughing and the fist that he made, which he believes to be enough to cover his cough, is inches away from his mouth. Really? I will give partial credit to the guy who decided to lift his newspaper to sneeze into it. It partially blocked the particles from hitting anyone directly in front of him, but not those escaping to the sides, top, or bottom of the newspaper. Unfortunately, it can't stop the airborne particles.

I've been writing this book off and on for years. I keep finding something new to say on the subject. I have a compromised immune system due to multiple sclerosis, so I can get sick easily. However, I've learned a lot over the years about how to stay well, how to protect myself when I go out, what to do when I am sick, and how to find alternatives for things when I can't go out. I want to share what has worked for me, so I can help others. I also want to drive home the fact that when you're sick and you expose yourself to people with compromised immune systems, it can have immense consequences for them, sometimes even death! It's true! Earlier this year, while writing this book, a friend of mine died of the flu. I can't help but think if he hadn't been exposed, he wouldn't have caught it and he wouldn't have died. I can't drive home that last point hard enough. Is it worth killing someone to go out when you're sick? It's something to think long and hard about. If you find it hard to care about a stranger, think about how you wouldn't want to get your family member, loved one or friend sick. What would feel if they were compromised in this way? Or if one of your loved ones died because of a contagious germ?

My mission is to keep the world well by starting a health etiquette movement! We need to start taking care of ourselves and others. If we're more proactive about health etiquette, fewer people will be sick, because we're not spreading germs around. I know this book is based upon staying home when you're sick, but it's also about staying away. Stay away from people you know are sick, unless you're a caregiver. If it's a spouse, partner, or parents, you can limit your time around them, while you both practice good health etiquette. Sleep in different rooms, if possible, to make sure you don't get sick and that you're getting proper sleep, if you're a light sleeper and their coughing would keep you awake. Why would you knowingly expose yourself to illness? In this instance, I'm talking about meeting up with sick friends, co-workers, etc. Encourage them to stay home and practice good health etiquette to prevent spreading their illness to others.

The good news is this book will help you to stay well, give you alternatives for going out, explain how to protect yourself and others when you do go out, and help you to understand the cycle of sickness. The bad news is that not everyone is going to read this book, stay home when they're sick or practice health etiquette. It's not my intention to shame you. My goal is to help you to understand the ramifications of going out when you're sick, how to prevent spreading your illness to others when you do have to go out, and how to stay well when you're around sick people.

2022 Version – Introduction

I have come full circle, as I'm on the train and looking at the handful of people who aren't wearing masks, despite it being required. These are the same people who didn't cover their mouths, prior to the pandemic. I also worry, as the restrictions loosen, that people will become reckless again, especially young college-aged people. They were having parties during the pandemic! As a result, they spread the virus to so many people, killing some of them. It also got them kicked out of college. I will say it again, "Is it worth killing someone to go out when you're sick?" I personally know a lot of people who have died due to COVID-19.

Some of my suggestions in Chapter 3, "Ways to Stay Well or Get Well When You're Sick" are pre-pandemic advice. In this 2022 version, I have added notes and alternatives. I have also updated cleaning information to Chapter 2, "The Most Germ Infested Places and Things You Can Clean" and a couple of other additions throughout the book. With the updates, now the book is applicable for any situation – pre-pandemic, pandemic, or post-pandemic.

People not staying home, not wearing masks, poor cleaning and hygiene practices are part of the reasons why this pandemic has lasted so long. In New Zealand, they were able to successfully contain the outbreak of COVID-19, due to their strict practices. I realize they're a smaller country, but it speaks volumes of what they were able to accomplish. I wish we had taken it more seriously in the United States and Europe.

I hope after the pandemic is over, people and companies will continue to be vigilant in their cleaning/hygiene practices. We need to continue to adopt a precautionary, preventative, and proactive approaches. I hope restaurants will continue using contactless menus, etc. And that businesses will adopt working from home for their current and future employees. It proves that disabled people can work from home.

But most importantly, remember the ***rule of thumb*** – If you're sick, stay home! And mask up if you must go out. Don't spread whatever you have, COVID or not, to a group of people. That's why COVID, the flu, etc. get out of hand. I'm not saying you have to wear a mask all the time. Just when you're sick or in certain situations, especially when mandated. Also, it's important to test if you have symptoms, but they're not always accurate, so use common sense and stay home and masked until your symptoms are gone. Too many people have depended on false results and end up testing positive later. Meanwhile they've spread it to so many people. Maybe realizing how many people have died of COVID-19 will drive home the message that people should be more compassionate and considerate of not spreading their germs, especially to the elderly and others with compromised immune systems. I have hope for the future. I think people are in a more receptive place to hear this message, especially because of the pandemic. At the same time, it breaks my heart to see the amount of apathy and misinformation contaminating our world. I wish more people had read my book prior to the pandemic. If you're reading this for the first time, this book will empower you to stay well!

1

THE SCIENCE OF SICKNESS

One of the best ways to prevent an illness is to be educated about it. In this chapter you will learn how you catch an illness, what its duration is, and how long you'll be contagious. When I say, "you" I mean yourself, your spouse, partner, children, grandchildren, parents, and other relatives and friends. When you know that, you can make the best decisions about when you are safe to leave home and when you are NOT safe to leave home, aside from seeking medical care, especially if you have one of the illnesses listed below.

The Top Illnesses YOU MUST NOT Spread

in no particular order

Meningitis

Meningitis is most commonly a serious viral or bacterial infection that affects the brain and spinal cord. Generally, it is spread through coughs, sneezes, and kissing or by being exposed to someone who has it, at home, school, or work. Although, there are several other rare ways to contract it. Meningitis is an inflammation of the meninges, the membranes that surround your brain and spinal cord.

It usually starts out like the flu with a fever or headache. However, the most tell-tale sign of meningitis is a stiff neck with a severe headache and fever due to the swelling of the membranes. The swelling is caused by inflammation. (If you see an illness ending in "itis" it means inflammation.) You often hear about meningitis outbreaks at colleges because students live in close quarters and often share food and drinks. As a general rule, do not share food and drinks with anyone.

Streptococcus

Strep is short for streptococcus, which is a common bacterium. It can be very hard to differentiate between a regular sore throat and strep throat. Some ways that you can tell it's strep are if you have a high fever (over 101°F/38°C), see red or white spots on your throat, have a skin rash, or a bad headache. One or more of these could indicate strep.

It is imperative to seek medical care for strep, because if left untreated, it can damage your heart (rheumatic fever) and kidneys. It can be very serious. My aunt got rheumatic fever from strep and she had to have a heart valve replacement.

Influenza

Flu, short for influenza, is a common virus. There are different strains, various countries of origin, and different viruses. The contagious period is also longer than that of other illnesses.

The name of the flu varies by where it originates. In 1989, it was called the Shanghai flu. My whole family caught it that Christmas. Everyone survived it, but decades ago, the flu killed millions of people. The biggest flu pandemic was in 1918, and it lasted for 2 years. Children, the elderly, pregnant women, and people with compromised immune systems can die from the flu. My friend's baby died in utero because she caught the flu. That's why I am so passionate about teaching others the consequences of going out when sick. Many lives are impacted.

Norovirus

Norovirus is a nightmare! It's the stomach and vomiting "bug." It is so highly contagious! According to the Journal of Medical Virology (2008), "Just a very small amount – as few as 18 viral particles – of norovirus on your food or your hands can make you sick. That means the amount of virus particles that fit on the head of a pin would be enough to infect more than 1,000 people!"[1] Cruise ships, schools, daycare centers, and nursing homes are the most common locations of the outbreaks.

The norovirus is spread through feces and vomit, which is why I am so strict about washing my hands, especially in a public restroom! To get rid of norovirus, wash your hands vigorously for 20 seconds under running water. Make sure to scrub under your fingernails, too. You can contract it by touching anything with the norovirus on it, by eating or drinking contaminated foods or drinks, or it may also be airborne. Do not prepare food for others when you have it either.

Speaking of food, be sure to wash fruits and vegetables well when you get them home from the grocery store. Be careful! Even shellfish can be contaminated. How many times have said you had food poisoning? Oftentimes, it is the norovirus and not any of the other viruses, bacteria, or parasites.

You're contagious for 2 weeks or even longer after you're feeling better, so people who feel better often go out right away and then spread it to others. This is especially common for babies in daycare and children in schools, as they do not stay away from daycare or

---

[1] https://www.cdc.gov/vitalsigns/norovirus/infographic.html

school that long. So proper handwashing is always essential, but especially after using the bathroom or changing diapers. And don't count on hand sanitizers, as they do not protect against norovirus. Be sure to wash the contaminated clothes carefully. Instructions are in Appendix 1. I could write a whole chapter on this!

Chickenpox

Chickenpox is highly contagious! If you are reading this, you have probably already had chickenpox, or you've had the vaccine, so this one especially relates to children and grandchildren.

Chickenpox causes blisters to break out all over the body. Cover the blisters to avoid spreading it to others, especially people with weakened immune systems, babies and pregnant women. Wash your and the child's hands thoroughly after touching the blisters. Once the blisters are crusty, they are no longer contagious.

In addition, shingles is a viral infection caused by the same virus that causes chickenpox. Anyone who has had chickenpox can see it reactivate as shingles years later. It's most common in people over 50 years old. Shingles causes a very painful rash. It is also contagious, and people with shingles can cause someone who is not immune to it to get chickenpox.

Pertussis

Whooping cough, or pertussis, is a bacterial infection of the respiratory tract. Many people get a harsh hacking cough, and the gasp or "whoop" that you make by breathing in, gave it its nickname.

The coughing is unlike that of any cold or flu, although it may start out feeling the same way. The coughing fits are so violent, they can make you vomit. It's also highly contagious and can be fatal for babies. That's why you must not spread this around! You're contagious for up to three weeks, and the coughing can last for months! At least 5 days of antibiotics do stop the contagion.

Tuberculosis

Tuberculosis (TB) is a very serious infection that affects your lungs. It also has a very violent cough that can cause you to cough up blood. It can be very painful. TB has other symptoms like fatigue and fever and can affect other parts of your body, such as the spine or the kidneys. It can really cause a lot of problems when it's active. My grandmother had TB and one lung collapsed due to experimental treatment for it.

TB is caused by an airborne bacterium, and you catch it by breathing in airborne droplets from coughs and sneezes. Not everyone with TB gets sick, though. Some people may be walking around with the latent TB. They carry the germ, but don't have symptoms. The only way to be sure of having it or not is by a skin or blood test. It's important to be tested. My father had the latent kind and had to take preventive medication.

Respiratory Syncytial Virus

RSV (Respiratory Syncytial Virus) is a common respiratory virus that causes mild cold symptoms in adults, but can be dangerous and deadly to infants, young children and adults with compromised immune systems, COPD, etc. If you have cold symptoms, stay away from infants and young children. Thousands are hospitalized and die every year due to RSV.

COVID-19

COVID-19 is a disease caused by the SARS CoV-2 virus that causes typical cold and flu-like symptoms such as a cough, fever, chills, aches. It ranges from mild to severe complications, including death. As of writing this, over 6 million people have died worldwide and 984,000 of that is from the United States! The way things are going, it'll be over a million. The scariest part is you can be asymptomatic and spread it to so many people. That's why it's important to wear a mask and get vaccinated. And so that it will stop mutating and causing new variants. This is the #1 illness you must not spread!

There are three primary ways to contract an infectious illness from another person that is caused by bacteria, viruses, fungi, or parasites. They are airborne, contact and droplet. Airborne includes coughing, sneezing, talking, breathing, even the spray from a toilet! Contact includes from surfaces you touch like doorknobs, railings, electronics or from direct contact like sex, kissing, bodily fluid exchange. Droplet also includes airborne, but these are when they touch your mouth, eyes, and nose.

Of course, sometimes you can eat contaminated food. Some are also transmitted by insects or animals, like mosquito bites and bats.

Here is a short list of the most common illnesses and how long you're contagious for. If I did not list your condition, look it up on the internet. I encourage you to become fully informed.

- *Cold* ~ 5-7 days.
- *Flu* ~ 7-14 days; 8 days on average, longer if your immune system is compromised such as with children, the elderly or people with various diseases such as HIV or multiple sclerosis. You can be contagious a day before your symptoms start.
- *Strep* ~ 24 hours after starting antibiotics.
- *Norovirus or Rotavirus* ~ 2 weeks! Stay home for at least 3 days after the last vomit or diarrhea!
- *Meningitis* ~ If viral, 3-10 days; if bacterial, 7-14 days.
- *Whooping Cough* ~ 3 weeks or after 5 days of treatment with antibiotics.
- *Chickenpox* ~ From up to 2 days before spots appear to about 5 days after the first spots.
- *RSV* ~ 5-8 days. 4 weeks in immunocompromised individuals.
- *COVID-19* ~ 2-14 days after exposure, before symptoms arrive. 10 days on average, but up to as long as 20 days after symptoms start. You're no longer contagious when you've been fever free without medication for 24 hours. Continue to quarantine for 10 days to 2 weeks. This can change depending on the variant and new guidelines. Double check with your physician.

Obviously, not everyone can afford to stay away from work, especially teachers, or medical professionals, nor can children usually stay home from school for more than a couple days. When you do return, take the time to practice good health etiquette!

Be careful when you choose to use antibiotics, as they are being way overused! Antibiotics will not help you recover from a common virus or flu. Antibiotics are for bacterial/fungal infections only! People are becoming resistant to antibiotics from being on them too often, and a lot of the time, they're not even needed.

27

2

THE MOST GERM INFESTED PLACES AND THINGS YOU CAN CLEAN

Be sure to use an anti-bacterial wipe, sanitizer or wash your hands after touching these germ-infested items! Clean these areas, if you're able. The goal is not to turn you into a germaphobe, but to make you aware of your surroundings and what items may be contributing to you getting sick. I had to use a sanitizer just to get through this chapter! Just kidding! ;)

Hand Washing – Making a meal? Wash your hands. Went to the bathroom (you or your animals) or changed a diaper? Wash your hands. Handled dirty clothes? Wash your hands. Treated a wound? Wash your hands. Came in contact with chemicals? Wash your hands. Sneeze? Blew your nose? Wash your hands. When in doubt, wash your hands!

Steps To Clean Hands:

1. Use your sleeve or hand to turn on the *faucet. Wet your hands and then turn off the water with your elbow, to help the environment. Don't waste water.

2. Put soap on your hands from a pump soap or one of the automatic soap dispensers. Bar soap is not recommended unless it's a last resort.

3. Scrub hands for at least 20 seconds, getting soap on both sides of your hands, in between your fingers and underneath your fingernails. Here's a visual for you. – https://www.youtube.com/watch?v=cbX0xwKORjk

4. Use your elbow to turn the water back on and rinse well.

5. Use your elbow to turn the water off and pat dry with a clean towel. Rubbing can create little cuts in your hands.

*If you have a sink that has two faucet knobs, turn them on and off in different places, so you don't get the germs or dirt back on your hands. Or find a paper towel to do that.

For more information on approved cleaners for COVID-19, look on the CDC website (https://www.cdc.gov/coronavirus/2019-ncov/prevent-getting-sick/disinfecting-your-home.html)

HOME:

Entrance

Doorknobs – Think about how many times a day you touch a doorknob. It's important to spray the doorknob with sanitizing spray or wipes. Or clean it with a warm, soapy cloth and follow it with vinegar to kill most germs, and to stay non-toxic. Or one of the COVID-19 approved cleaners.

Shoes – Take your shoes off at the door. Walking around outside, in hospitals, workplaces, stores and more. Your shoes pick up dirt, bacteria, and chemicals that you don't want to bring home. In one study, shoes were found to carry nine different bacteria! Consider a pair of shoes or slippers you only wear inside. I have a pair of shoes that I only wear inside the house and then when I am in my room, I take off my house shoes and walk around in my socks. Don't forget to be sure to wash your hands after taking off your shoes or tying them.

Light Switches/Lamp Knobs – If we counted how many times we turn the lights on and off it would be a very large number. Be sure to clean them the same way you clean the doorknob.

Purse or Backpack – Putting your purse or backpack on the ground, seats, or floor, picks up a lot of germs. It's like stepping all over it. Whatever you do, do not put it on a public restroom floor! If you are able, put it in the washing machine or use a sanitizing wipe or spray often. Or, clean as you would the doorknob.

Kitchen

Avoid bleach when you can. It's harmful to human health. It may also be harmful to wildlife when it goes down the drain. Don't overuse antimicrobial soap, either, as it doesn't always do the job and may contain toxins. Avoid cleaners with triclosan. Instead, use vinegar, although it does not kill staph, it kills many germs like E. coli and meningitis. The acid in it kills about 80% of all germs. Hydrogen peroxide is a good disinfectant that is antimicrobial. Use concentrations of less than 3%. Soap and water do a lot, especially when you scrub which can break down certain kinds of bacteria. Follow it up with vinegar to kill 99% of what's left.

Sponge – Sponges can harbor so much bacteria! You should replace your sponge every few weeks. And in between, microwave a wet, not dry, sponge for two minutes. It kills viruses and bacteria like E. coli! Be sure there are no metals in the sponge or plastic scrubber. Be careful as the microwaved sponge will be very hot! Clean it every other day if you use it every day. Or you can soak it in vinegar for five minutes, then rinse. The dishwasher also kills 99.9% of all germs, but make sure to use the heated dry setting.

Cutting Boards – Use the cutting board for vegetables and fruits. However, if you are cutting meat, use a plate or a plastic cutting board, so you can clean it in the dishwasher. Wooden cutting boards absorb bacteria quicker than you can clean them. Clean with vinegar to disinfect wooden surfaces you use for cutting fruit, veggies, or breads, or any wooden surfaces in your home. After using vinegar, you can use hydrogen peroxide on a wooden board to also kill germs!

Countertops – There are so many things that touch the surface of the countertops; from meat juices to money! Damp dishcloths harbor germs, so make sure they dry out thoroughly between uses. Be sure to wipe down the countertops nightly with a safe-around-food sanitizing cloth or spray with vinegar and wipe with a damp cloth, if it's not marble. If your countertops are granite, make sure they are sealed. Then it will be resistant to bacteria. You can clean it with a 50/50 solution of water and 91% isopropyl alcohol.

Kitchen Sink – A lot of things go in your sink; food, including meat juices, dirt from vegetables, etc., dirty dishes, soap residue, germs and dirt from washing your hands, and more. Be sure to clean it with hot water and soap. The other thing I do is combine baking soda and vinegar on the surface, on the strainer and down the drain. It also cleans the pipes. It kills E. coli, salmonella and many viruses! The combination of baking soda and vinegar is a fun thing for kids to watch, because the combination of the two makes it bubble and fizz.

Cabinets/Drawers – Make sure to clean anything that has a handle or knob. Make a spray bottle of a 1:1 vinegar and water solution. Use ½ cup vinegar and ½ cup water. Add 12-24 drops of an essential oil such as lemon or tea tree. Tea tree oil even kills black mold, and it smells good, too! Or one of the COVID-19 approved cleaners.

Refrigerator/Freezer/Stove/Oven - How many times have you felt a sticky refrigerator or freezer door handle? Food often splatters on the stove knobs. Make sure to clean them, too. To clean the refrigerator, remove the food and put it in a cooler until you're done. Remove drawers and shelves. Soak in warm soapy water or put in the dishwasher. Use baking soda paste on stubborn stains. Spray the inside of the fridge with your vinegar-and-water solution, soak and wipe down.

Microwave – Be sure to wipe down or spray disinfectant on the front door and buttons and be sure to clean the inside from splattered food, especially on the roof, and bacteria on the turntable glass plate. Put the glass plate in the dishwasher or wash it by hand. To loosen splatters, fill a microwave-safe bowl with 1 cup water and a chopped-up lemon (or 2 tablespoons lemon juice) with ¼ cup of vinegar until it boils. Let the bowl cool for 15 minutes before you open the door. A toothpick added to the water and vinegar can prevent the water mixture from exploding. If t's greasy, use a 50/50 water and vinegar solution on the glass window. Be careful not to damage the rubber gasket and use plain water to clean it or check the manual for other options. When you clean the outside, don't get cleaner in the vent holes. You might damage the inner workings.

Trash Bins/Cans – The resting place for all your trash! There are piles of germs – food, tissues, napkins, diapers (if applicable), and more!

Always line your bin with a bag. If you don't, please wash and sanitize it weekly. Wear rubber gloves if it's at all nasty. Remove contents. Take outside and hose it down completely, or do it in the shower, before you clean the bathroom. Use your vinegar-and-water spray to disinfect. Keep a special long-handled brush to scrub it with, and then clean the brush before you put it away. Throwing it in the dishwasher works well. Rinse and dry.

Water Bottles –

- Stainless steel bottles have several pros and cons. Normally, they last longer than glass or plastic bottles because steel bottles are corrosion resistant, meaning that they don't oxidize when exposed to sun or heat. Additionally, stainless steel is 100% recyclable. Stainless steel bottles are sometimes lined with a resin layer which can leach BPA. When buying a steel bottle, look out for a golden orange layer on the inside of the bottle which means that it's lined with BPA-epoxy.

- Glass is another option when choosing bottles. Although glass may not leech when left out in the sun, the recycling rate is much lower than plastic. Some public places also ban glass, and the cost of a glass bottle is typically higher than steel and plastic.

- Plastic looks to be the most popular water bottle. Plastic bottles are cheaper than stainless steel and glass bottles. But plastic bottles take nearly 700 years before they start to decompose. Additionally, plastic bottles leach in the heat.

- Bottle mouthpieces that are made of silicone seem to have no negative effect on health. It's probably safer than BPA-free plastic, but it may be hard to find.

- In many conditions like multiple sclerosis, autism, and Alzheimer's disease, aluminum already accumulates in the body, especially in the brain. Scientists are still researching what the impact is, but in the meantime, it's best to avoid aluminum exposure. (*By Isabel Zhang and Kolya Lynne Smith*)

Bathroom

Toothbrush – Our mouths are so dirty! Billions of bacteria live in your mouth at any given time! Therefore, it's very important to replace your toothbrush every couple of months and after you've been sick with the flu, strep or other illnesses. Rinse your brush before and after use. To store your toothbrush in-between uses, put it upright, handle down in an open holder. Let it dry thoroughly as that alone kills many bacteria. There are also UV devices that kill germs on your toothbrush.

To minimize germs in the bathroom, please make sure that you are flushing the toilet with the seat down. A small number of germs go airborne when you flush. Keep your toothbrush 2-3 feet from the toilet and close the lid before you flush.

Bathtub/Curtain – Mold, soap scum, fungus, athlete's foot, ring around the tub! A dirty shower curtain from bumping into it. I am mindful of not to do that, but if I do, I spray it down with vinegar solution. Avoid chlorine bleach since it's a known carcinogen and can cause burns, or gastrointestinal and respiratory problems. Oxygen bleach or hydrogen peroxide is a good disinfectant. Or, try vinegar, lemons and baking soda, as well as tea tree oil.

- Make a paste with ½ cup vinegar and ¼ cup baking soda to scrub bathroom tiles.

- For a multipurpose cleaner, make a spray that is 1/3 vinegar, 1/3 baking soda, and 1/3 water.

Bar of Soap – It seems like a bar of soap will not make you sick, but the truth is they carry a lot of germs. Especially if you've got soil, oil, etc. on your hands. Now you have black, dirty soap! The next time you go to wash your hands, you're using the same bar to get clean. If you have no other choice, run it under hot water until the dirt is washed or melted off. Instead, choose a liquid soap in a pump bottle or the best option, a motion-activated soap dispenser. Don't refill from a larger container but replace the bottle when it empties. Skip the washcloth, too, as it is a great place to breed germs. Use a facial brush on your face and let it dry thoroughly between uses.

Loofah Sponge – This mesh makes its way around your body more than your mate! It has soap residue built up in it, whether you rinse well or not. Be sure to replace it often! To minimize germs, dry it daily. Don't use after shaving for 2-3 days, as bacteria enters your skin through any nicks. Don't use on your face or genitals. Replace once a month. Better yet, consider not using a loofah, as it can grow staphylococcus germs and more.

Toilet – I call it the *"bowl of bacteria."* Always be sure to flush with the cover down! And when you go to clean it, start on the outer rim and then inner rim. If there are any spots of feces, clean that separately and spray it into the bowl with the cleaner. In-between cleaning, use a disinfecting spray. Clean the toilet before you get in the shower, so you always have a clean toilet to come back to.

White vinegar disinfects and eliminates odors. Borax (not boric acid) whitens, deodorizes, and removes stains. It is not toxic in small amounts. Lemon juice or citric acid can help get rid of tough stains. Tea tree oil kills most bacteria. Baking soda scours and deodorizes, though it doesn't kill germs.

Clean the toilet – let it soak with ½ cup of vinegar for a few minutes, or up to an hour if you have hard water. Brush and flush. Or to remove stains, try repeating the vinegar soak. It kills germs, bacteria, and mold. Try a hydrogen peroxide-based bleach for stain removing.

Check out Mindful Momma's idea for fizzy toilet bombs to use between scrubs (http://mindfulmomma.com/fizzy-toilet-bombs/).

Bathroom Sink – Clean handles daily, as they are teeming with germs. Whether you have one handle or two, use a tissue, your elbow, sleeve, or use a different spot to turn it on and or off, so your newly washed hands don't touch a dirty handle. Be sure to wash your sink often to get rid of soap scum, toothpaste residue, spit, and more. Use hot water. Wash it with a clean cloth or sponge. Rinse well with hot water, Spray it down with your cleaner of choice, such as the tea tree oil and vinegar solution. Scrub and wipe well. Use baking soda to scrub tough stains. Sprinkle on a dry sink, then scrub with a damp sponge or cloth. Don't forget to scrub the handles and faucet! Try an enzyme solution that eats through clogs for clearing the drain.

Makeup – Always make sure that your hands and face are clean before applying makeup. I suggest using your newly washed fingers as opposed to a wedge, that could harbor a lot of bacteria, unless you wash your sponges and brushes often! A woman I know got a staph infection from a dirty brush! If you have a cold sore, avoid using lipstick or use your finger to dab it on, saving the area where your cold sore is, until the last. Conjunctivitis is a common infection with your eye makeup! Avoid makeup when you're sick! Also, skip the makeup testers at the stores. You never know who have been handling them. Make a little bottle of alcohol to spray it on your makeup, use a cotton swab dipped in alcohol to clean them or alcohol pad.

Bedroom

Bed –

- Sweat, urine, feces, dust mites, bed bugs. Change linen often. Normally, a mattress can last 7-10 years; depending on how it is designed and how it is taken care of. Mattresses collect dead skin, body oil, and dust mites. A typical mattress can have as many as 10 million microscopic bugs.

- To take the best care of your bed, first invest in allergen-proof bed sheets. The sheets have fabric that is more tightly woven compared to regular sheets and prevent dust mites from separating from your mattress. If you're in a college dorm or low-income housing, get a bed bug incasement. Additionally, wash your sheets every week to two weeks at most. Washing sheets gets rid of most oils, dust, and dead skin. Vacuum your mattress often, too. Use a HEPA filter to collect dust from your bed. HEPA filters capture dust mites, pollen, pet dander, as well as many other things.

- Pillowcases also collect oils and dirt. I suggest swapping out your pillowcase every time you wash your sheets. People who struggle with acne might consider this helpful. *(By Isabel Zhang and Kolya Lynne Smith)*

Dresser – Dust and if necessary, wipe down the top. Wipe down the knobs or handles.

Clothing – Clothes get dirty for a lot of reasons, including sitting on surfaces that are dirty, like on the subway or hospital, food or drink stains, sweat, etc. But the dirtiest is underwear!

Wet Laundry – Just because it's been rinsed a few times doesn't mean that it's fully clean. That happens with the heat in the dryer or from the sun, which has ultraviolet radiation. Don't let wet clothes sit in the washing machine for a long time, before putting them in the dryer or outside (unless you have allergies to pollen). You could use bleach in your load to kill germs, but some have skin sensitivities or the clothes that are in the wash cannot withstand bleach. Every month or so, mix water and bleach, without any clothes and run the washing machine, to kill the germs in the washing machine drum. Always wash your hands after handling laundry – dry or wet. See the chapter, "The

Science of Sickness" for instructions on how to clean laundry with norovirus.

Computer – Keyboards can carry a lot of germs from your hands. Use a disinfecting cloth for your keyboard and mouse. Make a solution of 50/50 white vinegar and distilled water. Turn off the computer and unplug it for safety. Get a special vacuum attachment made for computers to vacuum out any crumbs and dust. Use a solution that is 50/50 vinegar and water and add a few drops of tea tree oil for its antibacterial effect. Dampen the cloth, not the computer, and wipe it down thoroughly. Make sure you've squeezed the cloth out, so it doesn't drip into the keyboard. Use a soft, dry cleaning cloth on the monitor. A microfiber cloth may take off fingerprints and other dirt. Dampen it with distilled water or to disinfect, 50/50 vinegar/distilled water. Apply cleaning fluid to the cloth, not the screen,

Living Room

Phone (Landline or Cell) – This is one of the most germ-infested items! Think about it for a second. Unless you are talking on a Bluetooth, it's pressing up against your face. Dialing, swiping, tapping with our fingers, that aren't always clean. We're taking it with us in the car, at work, school, on the subway, even in the bathroom, as we sit on the toilet (which you should avoid!), and more germ filled places! But luckily, just like with toothbrushes, there are devices that clean phones with ultraviolet light! As far as your landline, make sure to wipe it down with a sanitizing wipe (homemade or other). Make sure it's 70% alcohol or less. Don't use hand sanitizer, vinegar, window cleaner, bleach, or soap to clean your phones.

Remotes – Just like phones, these are germ-infested. Channel surfing with hands that aren't always clean. If the surface that they're resting on are not clean, that adds to it. Sometimes food particles or drinks fall on it. Be sure to wipe down your remotes often.

Furniture – Sitting on them with dirty clothes, sweat, dead skin, dust mites. Be sure to beat with a carpet beater often. I know you're picturing your grandmother in the backyard beating the carpet on the clothesline. Or you can use a hand-held vacuum. Then use disinfectant spray to clean and kill dust mites. If you want your fabric to smell good at the same time, spray some lavender, which is a deterrent.

OUTSIDE OF THE HOME:

Shopping

Money – Where has your money been? Who has touched it? Is there gas, oil, dirt, bodily matters, bacteria (staph), viruses (especially the flu), and even drugs (like cocaine) on it?! I used to count the money for a Bingo night. I was always careful to wash my hands thoroughly afterwards and I avoided touching my face, mouth, or eyes, before I washed my hands. To clean bills, put them in a mesh bag made for delicates and throw the paper money through the wash with a load of towels or jeans. Soak dirty coins in soapy water for 10-30 minutes, rinse thoroughly. Set to dry on a soft towel. Remember, cleaning coins removes the patina so if you are a coin collector, don't do it!

Gas Pump – Besides the obvious, gas, the handle can also harbor bacteria, viruses, diseases and more. The gas pump is dirtier than a toilet seat![2] The card reader and buttons are equally germ-infested, too. The germs are linked to food poisoning and other infections. Use an anti-bacterial wipe and sanitizer on your hands, keys, and anything else you might have touched after pumping! And wash your hands with soap and water when you get to your destination.

---

[2] https://www.ecowatch.com/gas-pump-germs-2013849186.html

Vending Machine – Would you like germs with that chocolate bar or bag of chips? Think of how many hands have reached into the bin where your food lands! Clean your hands before noshing!

Escalators – The railings of the escalator are loaded with bacteria, viruses, bodily fluids, etc. I've seen people sneeze right on the railing, while at the mall. Be sure to use hand sanitizer after you ride and avoid touching your face until you do. Here's something new! The company LG has come out with a UV light device for escalator handrails![3] I love it! But of course, they're not installed everywhere.

ATM/Cash Register Card Readers – This is another item that beats out the toilet for the most germ infested! Think of how many fingers have touched those keys in one day![4] Clean your hands after using one.

Office

Elevator buttons – What flora? Err, floor? Clean your hands after you ride!

Coffee Pot – The number of germs on the communal office coffee pot would give you a jolt, stronger than that of the caffeine! Bring your

---

[3].https://www.techspot.com/news/70158-lg-uv-sterilzer-escalator-handrails-germaphobe-dream.html

[4].http://abc7ny.com/health/are-nyc-atms-really-as-gross-as-you-think-they-are/1613751/

own coffee to work. If you do use the communal coffee pot, clean your hands before you sit down to enjoy!

Refrigerator – Not only do they steal lunches, they steal your health, by spreading bacteria and viruses. Use an ice pack in your lunch bag and keep it at your desk. There are insulated freezer lunch bags that keep food cold for hours.

Microwave – See above.

Stapler, Copier, Scissors, Pens, Pencils, Pencil Pouch - Use your own, or clean your hands after using shared equipment.

Computer – See above.

School

Water Bubbler or Fountain – It's like sharing a water bottle with thousands of people. A study showed that toilet water was cleaner than the water in the bubbler![5] Eww! Bring your own water bottle!

Desk – Whether you're at the same desk every time or if you move from classroom to classroom, you're coming into contact with even more germs! Clean it was you would anything else you touch. See above on making your own germ-killing cleaners.

---

[5] https://abcnews.go.com/GMA/story?id=3293080

Bathrooms – One of the worst bathrooms I've seen was when I was at college. I saw feces smeared against the wall! Can you imagine? For the most part, public restrooms are not harmful to your health. Make sure to clean your hands well after you use one.

Cafeteria Trays – Today's menu – Bacteria, with a side of viruses and bodily matter. Luckily, a lot of cafeterias have the cardboard trays. Plastic trays are laden with germs. Use plates under your food, even if you bring the food from home. Cover the tray with a napkin, too.

Entertainment

Amusement Park – Handlebars, seats, turn styles, bathrooms, food stands, etc.

Water Parks – This is frightening! There are so many things to come in contact with, at a water park – bacteria, viruses, foot fungus, bodily matters! And despite the amount of chlorine in the water, it doesn't prevent everything![6]

Beach – Another body of water that people use as a toilet! Add that in to the polluted water from litter, boats, chemicals, etc. and it's a health

---

[6] https://jezebel.com/water-parks-are-filthy-cesspools-of-despair-956061081

hazard! In 2017, beaches in Sydney, Australia were closed due to fecal matter in the water, because of rain storms the previous day.[7]

Zoo – Animals harbor a lot of germs! And if you're at a petting zoo, you come into direct contact with that. Not to mention the bathrooms and eating areas. Clean hands and teach your child not to touch his or her face until you've killed germs.

Playground – It's a playground for germs! Including MRSA, which is a serious bacterium! If you or your child get hurt at the playground, it can make things not so fun![8] Clean hands well after playing in the park.

Movies – Sticky floors (it's not always food/drink!), bathrooms, railings, seating for 1000's, and more! Clean your hands!

---

[7].https://www.nytimes.com/2017/01/02/world/australia/melbourne-beaches-storm-waste.html

[8] http://hvparent.com/playground-germs

Food

Restaurants – Menus have been found to be incredibly germ ridden. Hopefully restaurants will stay with the contactless menus. You place your order and then reach across the table for a roll! Condiments are touched by many different people over the course of a day. Some people ask for hot water to disinfect the utensils. If you order a drink, forego the lemon wedges, due to germs found in studies.[9] Buffets are also very dirty, between the handles and people coughing, sneezing, sometimes picking things up with their hands. Never take a plate from the top of the pile.

Groceries – Carts are handled by customers and sometimes workers. Wipe it down with the sanitizing wipe that most grocery stores offer. Of course, there's the card reader again. Also, shelving can be a hazard! I've gotten a cut from them before. Keep a first aid kit handy with Band-Aids and ointment. Keep hand disinfectant in the car to use after you leave the store.

Transportation

Public Transportation – It's full of bacteria, viruses, dirt and more; from the poles you hold onto, to the seats you sit on. You can catch anything from pink eye to the flu. Always carry sanitizer and anti-

---

[9].https://www.huffingtonpost.com/2014/01/27/lemon-germs-wedges-restaurants_n_4659168.html

bacterial wipes with you. Avoid touching seats and poles, if you can. And those are just things you touch. As I mentioned earlier, people are sneezing and coughing all around you. If possible, switch seats. I always make sure I am at least 3 or 4 people away from people, although this is difficult during rush hour. And I always cover my mouth with a clean bandana when I hear someone coughing or sneezing around me (pre-pandemic), but now I always have a 3–4-layer mask or N95 on. Face coverings are currently required on all modes of transportation. I'd continue to wear one even after the pandemic is over.

Car/Taxi/Ride Sharing – Car door handles, dirty seating, steering wheel, sick drivers past passengers…cars are full of germs! Vacuum and brush upholstery. Wipe down surfaces with your homemade disinfectant. If you ride in someone else's car, wash your hands afterward and don't touch your face until you do. Remember to put the windows down unless it's raining, snowing or too cold. Face coverings are required on all modes of transportation. I'd continue to wear one even after the pandemic is over, especially being in such tight spaces.

Airplanes – It's not just the air re-circulating, unless you happen to be on a newer plane that have HEPA filters, it's also the tray tables, seats, seatbelts, bathrooms, sick passengers and flight attendants! You're more likely to get sick from someone sitting near you. Clean your hands, use an anti-bacterial wipe on the tray table, take your own pillow and throw. Airports are equally germ-infested. Face coverings are required on all modes of transportation. I'd continue to wear one even after the pandemic is over, especially being in such tight spaces.

Trains – Similar to the public transportation subway, but add in the ticket agent, stubs, bathrooms, sick passengers, and agents. And if it's big enough, even the beverage/food areas. Use sanitizer and wash your hands when you arrive at your destination. Face coverings are required on all modes of transportation. I'd continue to wear one even after the pandemic is over, especially being in such tight spaces.

Ships – As mentioned in other chapters, cruise ships can be a port for norovirus, and now COVID-19. An acquaintance worked on a ship and talked about shaking so many hands, holding onto the railings, casinos, people handling the food at buffets, and more. Face coverings are required on all modes of transportation. I'd continue to wear one even after the pandemic is over.

Health

Hospitals – This is one place you can be guaranteed expose to bacteria and viruses, whether it's walking down the halls, in a crowded doctor's office, eating at the cafeteria or being in the ER. Masks are required in all health settings.

Nursing Homes – Norovirus outbreaks happen often, as well as COVID-19. I've seen loose stools in the bathrooms. There are also bacteria and viruses around. And those with bed sores can easily get infections, especially if they have dirty sheets or hands. There is also a lack of heath etiquette in elderly. I've seen feces and dirt underneath their nails. Another part of it, is losing their eyesight. Masks are required in nursing homes.

Gyms – Wipe down the equipment before and after you use it! And then there's the risk for fungus in locker room showers, floors, and dirty bathroom stalls. Face coverings are required at most gyms. It's a smart thing to do with everyone huffing and puffing during exercise.

Restrooms (Anywhere!) – Use your elbow, foot, clothing, etc. to open and close the door. Some people wash their hands after entering the bathroom. You can imagine the number of germs on the soap dispenser and toilet seats, especially portable toilets! (I refuse to use them.) If you're in a bathroom that uses hand dryers, pass it by. It sucks up fecal matter and then blows it on your hands! Carry a clean facecloth with you in your handbag or backpack.

3

WAYS TO STAY WELL OR GET WELL WHEN YOU'RE SICK

Prevention plays a big role in staying well. Too often, we don't take care of ourselves, until we've gotten sick. And even then, it's sometimes difficult, because we're so tired from the illness. I can guarantee that self-care will absolutely keep or get you well, than if you didn't take care of yourself at all.

Here are some ways to shorten an illness or prevent it all together:

Physical

Water – Staying well hydrated will help keep your nose moist, which is one of the main entrances for germs. I talk more about this below. Drink water slowly, to hydrate properly, otherwise it goes through you too quickly and your cells won't have time to absorb it, you'll end up peeing it out. For example, drink 1 cup, 4 times an hour. Also, if you drink it too fast, you risk losing sodium levels in your blood which can be dangerous.

Electrolytes – Be sure to drink an electrolyte drink if you've been sweating, having diarrhea or vomiting. Be careful to avoid those with a high level of sweeteners or artificial colors and flavors.

Lemon Water – Lemons contain a lot of Vitamin C which detoxifies the liver. They can also help ease nausea. The hot water also helps moisturize your nose, so you will breathe better.

Tea – Look into which herbal, black and green teas help you and try a few.

Vitamins/Minerals – Vitamin C and D3 are the best. Make sure to get your levels of Vitamin D tested before taking it. Zinc is an important mineral for your immune system.

Healthy Foods – Protein is important for a healthy immune system. Eat antioxidant rich foods. As well as anti-viral, anti-bacterial, and anti-microbial foods (search the internet for lists of these foods). Avoid dairy, wheat, sugar, fried foods, and drinking alcohol.

Turmeric – This herb as flu fighting properties. It is a powerful anti-inflammatory. Take it with black pepper for better absorption.

Ginger – Ginger is in the same family as turmeric. It's great for nausea, relieving a sore throat and much more! It's my go-to when I have a cold.

Other Herbs and Spices – Garam Masala has been shown to boost the immune system. I have containers of herbs and spices organized by specific categories; Anti-viral, anti-bacterial, anti-fungal, anti-inflammatory, anti-microbial (search the internet for lists of these foods).

Sleep – As a society, we are often sleep-deprived. Sleep plays a big role in keeping the immune system strong.[10]

Exercise – Take a walk around the block, work out in the gym, swim in the pool, ride your bike to work, kickboxing can get out a lot of

---

[10].https://www.mayoclinic.org/diseases-conditions/insomnia/expert-answers/lack-of-sleep/faq-20057757

frustrations, or whatever exercise you like best. Being sedentary lowers your immune system.

Sanitizer, Anti-Bacterial Wipes, Wash Hands – Often! Pat them dry, as opposed to rubbing your skin with a towel or rough paper towel, which can cause tiny cuts. Sanitizer is good in a pinch, but it doesn't remove dirt and bacteria (just viruses). For dirt and bacteria, use the anti-bacterial wipes. But they should never be a substitute for soap and water.

Avoid Touching Eyes/Nose/Mouth – If you have germs on your hands, you will pass them on, through your eyes, nose, or mouth. Clean hands often to limit spreading illness.

Cover Cuts and Wounds – Some people don't like to wear bandages, because they don't want to look juvenile, but there are clear options now, including liquid bandages that just cover the cut.

Bandanas And Masks –

Bandanas: 25x25 ideal, but 22x22 will work as well. Make sure the bandana fabric is thick. Some bandanas have a thin material, that won't block particles from coming through. Hold it up to the light after it's folded to be sure, or if it's packaged, lift one layer to see if it's thin material. You can also make a bandana out of your favorite fabric to ensure it's fashionable and thick enough.

Steps to fold your bandana:

1. Lay your bandana on a flat surface in a diamond shape.
2. Fold down, in half, so you make a upside triangle shape.
3. Then fold down again, the height of your nose and mouth. About 4.5 inches.
4. Tie your bandana around the nape of your neck.
5. Tuck the tail of the bandana into your shirt.

If you're not wearing a mask, a bandana around your neck provides a quick, easy way to cover your mouth, to both protect you from someone else and to protect them from your sneeze or cough. You do have to be careful when you go into certain places, like banks (pre/post-COVID). When that was the case, pre-pandemic, I covered my mouth with my sleeve, my hand or I lifted the collar of my shirt and covered my mouth, when wearing short sleeves. Don't constantly cover your mouth with the bandana. If you don't want to wear the bandana around your neck, keep it in your pocket to cover your cough or sneeze, or to cover your mouth and nose to protect yourself from someone else.

Masks: Some people wear the flimsy hospital face masks thinking that it will keep them well, but that doesn't work for airborne particles, unless you're wearing a specialized filtering mask. Here's a link to 10 most popular face masks.[11] The best mask to wear is an N95 (my favorite is the Gerson 3230 N-95, because it fits my face the

---

[11] https://themighty.com/2018/01/face-masks-brands-cold-flu-prevention/

best, with no gaps), KN95, if you can't find them or aren't comfortable for your face, look for a mask that's 3-4 layers thick (if you're able, insert a filter in your mask), adjustable behind the ears and has a nose clip. You want to make sure there's no gaps. I cringe every time I see someone's mask full of gaps, because it's not protecting them or you. I've seen people wear the hospital masks so low, that it's almost on their neck, and meanwhile their nose is being exposed when they speak. Wear it higher on the nose, to allow for any slipping that occurs. Another reason why it's best to wear a mask with a nose clip. Don't wear the same mask every day. Rotate them. Make sure you're washing your cloth masks after each use or wearing new N95's daily, rotate them (7 masks per week). They can be reused for a total of 40 hours of wear per mask. Depending on how long you wear them, on average, they'd last several weeks. Hospital face masks were designed to keep germs contained. It's very important to wear a good mask when you're sick and replace it often! Since hospital masks aren't effective in protecting what you're breathing in, a thick bandana, certain clothing, an N95, KN95, or a filtered face mask (3-4 layers) will help protect you from illness. I've been wearing face coverings for almost 6 years (2022) and I've avoided the flu, strep, colds, etc.

Another great tip is, if someone is coughing or sneezing, breathe out slowly or hold your breath, as you walk past them, and don't breathe in until you're far enough away to feel safe.

Nasal Rinse – You can use a Neti Pot (if you can tolerate it) or use saline mist. A dry nose catches germs because the hairs trap them just like a filter. So don't pluck your nose hairs, but you can trim them if necessary.

Nasal Gel, Petroleum Jelly, Aloe Vera, or Lotion Tissues – Use these for a raw nose and to keep your nasal passages lubricated. It is extremely important to use a nasal gel before going on a flight because of the extremely dry air. During the winter, use nasal gel throughout the day.

Hot Steam/Humidifier – Use a towel to create a tent. Don't lean over the stove but pour 4 to 6 cups of very hot water into a glass bowl. Add a few drops of peppermint, wintergreen, eucalyptus or a decongestant blend. You don't have to use boiling water but can use the hottest water that comes out of the tap. In fact, boiling water can do harm by burning you or overheating pores so lower the temperature! You could also take a hot shower and breathe in the steam. During the winter, it's important to use a warm mist humidifier to keep your nasal passages moist. Some humidifiers have a steam feature, instead of using a pot/ bowl or the shower.

Sweating – Sweat through exercise or a sauna. It detoxifies your body.

Air Purifier – Make sure you get one with a HEPA filter and a UV light that kills germs. Shop around on Amazon and other reputable stores. National Allergy Supply is a good online store.[12] The family who owns it has lots of experience and the company provides very good service. You can get safe cleaners, sheets, mattress covers, and more there, too.

Hugs/Touch – Get some daily! If you can't find someone, cuddle a pillow, use a weighted blanket, or give yourself a long hug, no shorter than 20 seconds! Heck! Go for 20 minutes! I suggest being held by someone or holding a pillow for 15 minutes straight, every day, or more. When you hug yourself or a pillow, think about someone you love. Your brain can't tell the difference between that and an actual hug from a loved one. It releases the same great chemicals. Touch is so important! It boosts your immune system and releases your love hormone, oxytocin, which reduces cortisol. I used to belong to a group of affectionate people. During the years I was with them, I got sick only twice in two years. When I stopped being around them, I was constantly getting sick. Those hugs had a big impact on my health! I'm currently working on a research paper on touch and the immune system. I started a touch therapy practice – Hold To Heal. I'll do virtual visits until the pandemic fades. For more information go to www.holdtoheal.com Note: Long, close hugs are not advisable, currently. Wearing masks is also important. Quick hugs are OK, if you hold your breath and when each of you turn your head in the opposite direction.

____

[12] https://www.natlallergy.com/

Pets – Animals are a great source of touch. Stroke a dog, cat, guinea pig, or other animal of your choice for 15 – 20 minutes to reduce your blood pressure, anxiety, and depression. It also boosts your immune system.

Massages – Massage boosts your immune system by relieving stress, increasing circulation, and draining the lymphatic glands. Note: Massages are now approved with masks in some locations.

Medicine – I try and stay away from medications if I can. Side effects often do harm, and the combinations of them need to be carefully checked. Use an online drug checker to be sure each new medication is safe to take.[13] I don't take a fever reducer unless it's over 101. There's nothing like a cold washcloth. I have fond memories of my Gram putting them on my forehead. There are so many home remedies that help, just as effective, like steam, saline washes, honey, saltwater gargling, and more. People who take decongestants for their nasal symptoms are doing more harm, because sneezing and blowing your nose gets rid of the germs, but decongestants dry your nasal passages. Take the medications you deem necessary but research each one to check for safety and effectiveness. Search online for your symptoms with the word remedy or homeopathic or alternative to find other options.

Mental/Emotional

---

[13] https://www.drugs.com/drug_interactions.html

Relax – Stress is bad for your immune system. When you're stressed, your body produces cortisol. Too much in your system affects your immune system and frankly, your entire body. In 2015, I caught one illness after another, for 3 months, because I was so stressed. Stress less, by going slow. So often we rush through life. Mindfulness forces you to slow down and be aware.

Fun – Have fun! Act like a kid! As adults we tend to be too serious and be hyper focused on work, but we forget to play. We need to take the time every day to play! Research has shown that it's a time of creativity and ideas. Decide which kid-like activities you want to do and enjoy! It will boost your immune system.

Laughter or Laughter Yoga – Ha! Ha! Ha! Laughter improves the immune system, while decreasing cortisol. It also releases endorphins, which is one of your chemicals that makes you feel good. If you're already sick, you want to do this at home, so you don't share your germs through your breath or droplets from laughing. Laughter is OK at a distance and with a mask on. Laughter Yoga is not advisable during COVID-19, flu season, etc.

Meditation/Spirituality/Prayer – There are countless research studies proving that meditation, spirituality and prayer helps promote healing.

Volunteering – Being of service and helping others makes you feel so good. All of the happy hormones; serotonin, oxytocin, dopamine and endorphins are released when you're volunteering! So many people are low on these hormones, which can cause fatigue, depression, brain fog, addictions, and more. You can overcome this naturally. If you can volunteer safely during the pandemic, do so. There are some organizations that are calling people via the phone or video chat to ease loneliness in the elderly and immune compromised individuals.

Socialize – Loneliness is an epidemic in our technology dependent and busy society. We can be with people and still feel lonely, so find your tribe. It definitely affects your immune system. We need connection and as I mentioned above, touch. One way to ease your loneliness is to visit the elderly, as they are widely affected by loneliness and touch deprivation. Please socialize safely with masks and social distancing indoors. Schedule most of your visits outdoors. If you're sick, make sure you schedule video chats and phone calls to stay connected.

Happiness/Positive/Gratitude – When you're happy and in a positive frame of mind and grateful heart, it can absolutely make you feel better and prevent you from becoming sick. Being fearful about becoming sick, could make you sick. Take care of your mind, as well as your body.

Self-Love/Self-Care/Self-Compassion – These are essential to overall health. Please love, care for, and be compassionate to yourself. There's a difference between self-love and self-care. You can take all the bubble baths you want, but if you're not loving, accepting or being kind to yourself, it won't help entirely. There are a lot of self-love/self-care/self-compassion books and websites out there to help you along this path.

Authenticity – Our bodies and minds can tell when we are not being authentic; if we're lying, hiding a piece of ourselves, or changing your behavior to please someone else, etc. Of course, there are times when we do have to do those things as a form of protection, but for the most part, do your best every day to be authentic and you will feel better for it!

65

4

PLACES PEOPLE GO WHEN SICK (AND ALTERNATIVES FOR THEM)

There are so many places that people go when they're sick, and it is just not necessary! Sick? Stay home! All it does is wear you out, when you should be recuperating, instead of spreading germs to others, and among those could be the people at high risk of catching an illness.

If it's a matter of not wanting to be alone, I understand. You can talk to friends on the phone, on the computer… there are so many ways today including messaging or video chat. If it's a matter of being bored, with the computer, phone, television, books and more, there are endless opportunities to be entertained.

A lot of people have difficulty being alone. They can't stand to stay in the house when they're sick. If you have cabin fever, step outside of your house where you won't come into contact with anyone. The fresh air will make you feel you good and cleanse your nose and lungs.

Here's a list of where people go when they're sick and some alternatives:

Food

Restaurants – You don't need to go out to a restaurant when you are sick. Being around food when you are sick is one of the best ways to spread your germs to a lot of people at once. Instead, order takeout or cook your favorite comfort food at home. Have some frozen or prepared meals on hand for times like these.

Coffee Shop – I know we all need our caffeine fix, but instead buy and freeze a bag of your favorite coffee. That way you can have a cup of good coffee within your reach anytime.

Bakery/Donut Shop – You don't need sweets when you're sick. Sugar worsens phlegm production. Focus on eating healthy foods. If you must get your sweet tooth fix, call a bakery have delivery service. Better yet, have something you already have at home.

Grocery Store – Grocery shopping is exhausting, and you don't want to be holding a tissue in one hand and pushing the cart with the other. Almost all grocery stores deliver now. Or use another food delivery service. Even services like Amazon have grocery sales. If you ask a neighbor, have them leave your bags on the front stoop and pay them when you're well.

Bar – Despite some wives' tales, drinking alcohol will not kill the germs to the point where you will recover. You cannot drink enough to make a difference without having alcohol poisoning! Alcohol may seem soothing, but it can dehydrate you, making you sicker. It may also conflict with medications you're taking and can worsen sleep apnea. For example, alcohol and Tylenol or Ibuprofen can damage your liver or stomach.

Ice Cream Shop – Ice cream slides down easily and feels good on a sore throat. It provides calories when eating may be difficult, but it can also make your throat swell more, due to the sugar in it. It thickens phlegm, irritating throats and making a cough worse. In addition, when you're sick, dropping your body temperature slows down healing. As a general rule, avoid ice cream when you're sick. Stick to juice pops and ice chips instead if you need a cooling alternative.

Entertainment

Movie Theater – Sure, it's a good distraction from your illness, but nobody wants to hear someone coughing or sneezing around them as they're trying to pay attention to the movie. All I can think about is that scene from the movie, "Outbreak!" There are plenty of streaming services or whip out when of the movies you own. Better yet, watch some home movies. Reminiscing makes you feel good, it boosts your immune system by activating your happy hormones – dopamine, oxytocin, endorphins, and serotonin

Comedy Club – While laughing raises your happy hormones, it can also cause you to go into a coughing fit! You do not want the comedian to use you as part of their skit! When you are sick, watch a funny movie, TV show, comedy sketch or play a silly game at home where you can benefit from laughing, but not disturb others or spread your germs.

Theater – Who done it? Who sneezed? Who coughed? When you're sick, give away your tickets and stay home. Just as there is health etiquette, there is also theater etiquette. Theater actors have to deal with enough already and having a sick audience member is one they'd like to avoid.

Concert – Stay home and blast your music as loud as you can (without damaging your eardrums)! If you have neighbors or someone else to disturb, use your headphones! Just don't go to the concert sick. Be kind to other music lovers!

Places of Worship

This is one of my biggest pet peeves! Whoever your highest power is, they will forgive you for not worshipping in a formal structure. When you're sick, you can do it on your own from home. Going when you're sick is almost sacrilegious or impious. You're exposing people to germs while they're connecting to their higher power, especially if you're hugging, kissing and shaking their hands! If you're still concerned about that, you can fold your hands (Namaste style), hold your hands out as if you were praying over them (which also doubles as "stay away from me") or put your hands over your heart. Would your higher power do this harm? No.

Work

Use one of your sick days. Don't use them up on days when you're not really sick. If you have the option, please work from home. If you MUST go to work, then make sure that you practice good health etiquette.

Shopping

Mall – You don't need to get those pair of shoes right away. Shop online. No lines and you get to do it in your pajamas!

Drugstore – Make sure that you have cold and flu supplies on hand. If not, have someone you know go buy them for you. Or get them delivered. Some places deliver the same day.

Schools and Daycares

Schools and daycares, attended by people of any age, are some of the most common places for spreading germs. Have a classmate get the homework assignments or find them online. Use email to check with your instructor.

Miscellaneous

Yoga – Attending class with a fever is not what they mean by hot yoga![14] Stay home and practice gently on your own.

Non-Emergency Medical Appointment – Such as physical therapy, acupuncture, chiropractor, or mental health appointments (do it over the phone or video chat). If you must go, then practice good health etiquette.

Bank – Don't "hold up" the tellers with your germs! Take advantage of online banking or use the ATM machine, remembering to wipe it down with sanitizer, after using. Or simply wait to do your banking until you're feeling better.

Beauty Salon – You don't need to get your hair, nails, or anything else done on your body when you're sick. Don't spread illness to your beautician.

Meditation – It's "Om!" not "Oh, oh!" as you cough and sneeze. No one can concentrate with someone coughing, sniffling or sneezing right next to them. Stay home and find guided meditations[15] or relaxing tunes on the internet.

---

[14] https://en.wikipedia.org/wiki/Hot_yoga

[15] http://marc.ucla.edu/mindful-meditations

Wakes or Funerals – Don't go to a wake or funeral sick. The last thing a grieving family and friends need is an illness to make them feel even worse. They will understand why you didn't come. Grief affects your immune system, so they're more vulnerable to illness.

Parties or Special Events – Cancel your plans when you're sick! Whether it's a baby shower, a birthday party or another event, it's not right to be around others when you're sick. They will understand, especially if it's a baby shower. The last thing the pregnant woman needs is to get sick. We already know that the flu can kill a baby in utero.

Transportation

Vehicles – If you take taxis and ride sharing services, consider waiting until you are well, or practice health etiquette, if you must go out. Drivers get annoyed at sick passengers. I had a great conversation with a ride sharing driver about this.

Planes, Trains, or Buses – Nobody wants to sit next to or across from someone who's sick, especially when they are in a confined space where you can't open a window or filter the air properly. Practice health etiquette or be kind and stay home.[16][17]

---

[16] http://www.health.com/cold-flu-sinus/germs-youre-more-likely-to-catch-on-public-transit-than-ebola

[17] https://www.insidescience.org/news/tracking-germs-planes-and-buses

If I didn't list the place that you're thinking of going, DON'T GO! STAY HOME! Find an alternative or do something else! You really need to cancel your plans, whatever they are, when you or your kids are sick. Don't drag your sick kids around with you, just because you want to go out.

5

DON'T BE GENEROUS WITH YOUR GERMS

Note: This chapter was written pre-pandemic (2018).

I was on the train when I saw a woman texting with both hands, so she didn't bother covering her cough! Ugh! Put the cell phone down and cover your mouth! I saw the same thing with a woman who was reading a book. It's lazy, rude, and so selfish! Has our culture become so apathetic and desensitized that we don't care about health etiquette? "Well, nobody else covers their mouth. Why should I? People go out when they're sick. Why shouldn't I?" These apathetic attitudes are why we're becoming sick more often! We need to care for ourselves and care about others! Have we become too busy to clean, too busy to wash our hands, to cover our mouths, to practice good health etiquette in general? Make the time! Health etiquette is a habit that we have to hone. Just like any other habit, we must make a conscious effort to practice it every day. Your health and others will thank you.

Being chronically ill, I've been in my share of emergency rooms and doctor's offices. "HAAAAAACK!" That's all I hear, every few minutes! Why is this person not wearing a mask? There is signage everywhere! One of the things that bothers me the most is the medical field not enforcing the rule that people wear masks when they're sick. Are they afraid they'll offend? They leave it up to the person. I've never seen a staff member ever go out to the coughing or sneezing accuser and tell them to put on a mask. I think people don't want to wear the medical masks because they feel embarrassed, they don't want attention drawn to them, that people will make assumptions or even that they don't look cool. People need to take precautions and choose protection over vanity!

COVER, COVER, COVER your MOUTH! We were taught as children to cough into our elbow, but this is all wrong! It's not a tight seal. Just as coughing into a fist is not a tight seal. The droplets/spray from the cough or sneeze can escape through the bottom or top of the elbow nook. Instead, cough into your shirt, sleeve, tissue, napkin, paper towel, bandana or your hand and wash your hands afterwards. It doesn't take that much effort to do it. When you cough or sneeze into your sleeve or shirt, use your hands to cover your mouth, to make sure it's a tight seal. Even if your cough or sneeze is from allergies or another non-contagious cause, cover your mouth anyway! No one wants to feel the breeze of a cough or sneeze or get drops of fluid on their face or clothing. A sneeze can travel at 39 miles per hour! Think about that!

WASH, WASH, WASH, WASH your hands! Wash vigorously in cold, warm or hot water and soap for at least 20 seconds, making sure to clean the front and back. I've seen people who only wash their fingertips with a dab of soap! Also, don't forget your nails. Wash your hands, especially after using the bathroom. I witness people all the time use a public bathroom, like at a hospital or movie theater, and leave without washing their hands! You shouldn't even do that at home, much less a public bathroom! I read feces can go through up to 10 layers of toilet paper, so you can probably double that number in public restrooms with thin toilet paper! I saw one woman in the hospital bathroom who had had an accident with her bowels. She was wiping herself at the bathroom sink, then she went back to the stall to finish and then she walked out of the bathroom without washing her hands! When you leave there, and you have her dirty hands on yours by touching the same doorknob. Unknowingly you have something to eat, believing your hands are already clean, because you washed them in the bathroom. But then you and hundreds of others come down with the norovirus. It's very contagious! You can be contagious for as long as two weeks! So please, wash your hands and wash often.

Don't pick your nose. Blow it or use a folded tissue to pick it. If you do pick it with your finger, wash it immediately or use sanitizer, if you don't have access to soap and water. Also, don't use a handkerchief or use the same tissue more than once. You get germs on your face and hands, by re-using the same area.

Be careful with your furry friends, too. Animals can catch your cold and flu.

Please remember that not everyone has a normal immune system. Those among us who at high risk for illness include those with cancer, AIDS, MS, cystic fibrosis, diabetes, the elderly, children, immune system disorders and more. Children haven't built up their immune system, so they get sick more often than adults. In the elderly, as they age, their immune system gets weaker and they're not strong enough to fight off the infections. And I'm concerned that even those without compromised immune systems are compromised because of being stressed, sleep deprived and eating poor diets.

Since children get sick the most often, it's very important to teach them proper health etiquette. Avoid play dates when they're sick.

In Washington State, you can get fined for giving someone a cold. It's a misdemeanor.[18] A word of caution if you live there!

I often think about how entire civilizations were wiped out because people brought diseases and illness to people who hadn't been expose to it before. For example, the Incas when the Spanish invaded or when Native Americans were exposed to "white man's" diseases and illnesses, such as smallpox, typhus, etc.

---

[18] http://www.nbcrightnow.com/story/37323965/going-out-in-public-with-the-flu-or-cold-you-could-actually-be-fined

79

6

COSTS OF SICKNESS

Work, Health Insurance, Missed Events, and More.

Note: This chapter was written pre-pandemic (2018).

A lot of people don't think about the costs of sickness, such as the cost of losing a day's pay (if you don't have paid sick days). Many cannot afford a day off from work. The worst is when food workers go to work sick! I bet you anything if people started suing companies for having sick workers, they'd change their policies for sick days. Find organizations in your state who advocate for paid sick days. Join them! You're not going to be a very efficient or productive company if half your office is out sick. It's estimated that the common cold causes around 25 billion annually in productivity losses. If health etiquette is practiced, you will reduce that number. Same thing goes for the classroom. It is never too early to start teaching and practicing health etiquette. Schools who encourage perfect attendance should not count sick days. I also understand that it's difficult for working parents to care for their sick children, but do not send them to school if you have another option of getting a babysitter or having them stay with someone else. I have heard of places called, "sick daycare" who specifically care for sick children who can't go to school.

Many people don't have health insurance. How much does it cost every year when people are sick? Some people are turning towards crowdfunding sites to help pay for their medical expenses. Medical bills have really gotten out of hand. Everyone should be able to afford health care. It should be a right, not just a privilege! So many people have become bankrupt due to medical expenses. In fact, it's the number one cause of bankruptcy![19]

I was scheduled to have surgery and when I was in the pre-op appointment waiting are there were a few sick people there. Two days later I was sick, and I had to cancel my surgery. Think about that for minute! That's serious! That's another reason why I'm so passionate about advocating that people stay home when they're sick. Another time, I had plans to go on vacation and I had to cancel because I got sick.

But, the ultimate cost, is when someone dies because they got sick! It happens all too often.

---

[19] https://www.cnbc.com/id/100840148

CONCLUSION

There's a tug of war that's going on these days. By going out when you're sick, you're spreading germs around to a lot of people. As a result, people are getting sick more often. If people stayed home, everyone would get sick less often, and nobody likes being sick. Unless we can get back to a place where we stay home when we're sick and practice health etiquette, it's only going to get worse. We'll turn into a constantly contagious community if we aren't already. Flu rates have skyrocketed, because people aren't staying home when they're sick and/or they're not practicing proper health etiquette. Look what happened with COVID! We need to learn this now, before the more complicated contagions like drug-resistant bacteria, Ebola, SARS, and most recently, COVID or unknown illness that hits us in the future, does its damage.

My primary goal of this book is to prevent people from getting sick, to lead healthier lives, to practice health etiquette and to stay home when sick. If people get sick less often, I've achieved my goal. If a life is spared, because a sick person stayed home, that would be the ultimate goal!

WHERE DO WE GO FROM HERE?

Thank you for reading this entire book; it's been years in the making. I hope that I have educated you on many things regarding illness such as places to avoid and clean, heath etiquette, and especially the importance of staying home when you're sick. Please spread the word about this book, to extend the gift of health to as many people as possible! And please consider leaving a review for my book.

Coming soon, I will be launching the adapted children's book version, "Wizard Of Well"

You can contact me at sickstayhome@gmail.com

Follow me at any of the following:

www.facebook.com/sickstayhome

www.instagram.com/sickstayhome

www.twitter.com/sickstayhome

www.pinterest.com/sickstayhome

sickstayhome.tumblr.com – Blog

APPENDIX 1: NOROVIRUS

Outbreak Management - Disinfecting Your Home

Noroviruses are a group of viruses that cause acute gastroenteritis in humans. The symptoms of norovirus infection include nausea, vomiting, diarrhea, cramping and low-grade fever. Noroviruses are transmitted through the fecal-oral route—either by consumption of fecally contaminated food or water, direct person-to-person spread, or environmental contamination. Norovirus is very contagious and can also be spread through tiny droplets of material in the air (aerosols).

Cleaning Procedures

If you or someone in your home has been exposed to and has symptoms of a norovirus, it is important to thoroughly clean and disinfect your living environment to prevent others from becoming ill. Preparation is important. Be sure to use disposable gloves, a mask, a form of eye protection and protective clothing while thoroughly cleaning. Keep children away from the area before cleaning and as you clean.

It is best to use chlorine bleach (sodium hypochlorite-NaOCl) as the main disinfecting agent (other types of disinfectants are not effective at killing the virus). Use a new, unopened bottle of chlorine bleach and prepare the cleaning solution as indicated below under "Concentrations," using fresh bleach each day. Discard unused portions. (Open bottles of chlorine bleach will lose effectiveness after 30 days, so use a new bottle of bleach every 30 days for accurate concentrations.) Warning: chlorine bleach may damage fabrics and other surfaces. Please spot-test the area before applying to visible surfaces.

Concentrations

- For stainless steel, food/mouth contact items: 1 tablespoon of chlorine bleach in 1 gallon of water.
- For non-porous surfaces such as tile floors, counter-tops, sinks, etc.: one-third (1/3) cup of chlorine bleach in 1 gallon of water.
- For porous surfaces such as wooden floors: one and two-thirds (1 2/3) cups of chlorine bleach in 1 gallon of water.

Leave the bleach solution on the surface for 10 to 20 minutes, and then rinse the area well with clean water. After the disinfection process is complete, close off the area, if possible, for at least one hour. If there are windows, air out the area.

Wash and sanitize hands thoroughly immediately after cleaning.

Cleaning Procedures for Special Cases and Areas

For areas exposed to vomiting or feces (poop) contamination:

- Use paper towels to soak up as much of the vomit or feces as possible, being careful not to drip or splash the material.
- Clean and disinfect the entire area with disposable cloths.
- Dispose of all waste material in sealed plastic bags.

For carpeted areas:

- Remove all visible contamination with paper towels or other absorbent material. Discard in a plastic bag to minimize aerosols; seal the bag and put in a garbage can.

- Steam-clean the carpet to 170 degrees Fahrenheit for five minutes or 212 degrees Fahrenheit for one minute to completely inactivate the virus.

For linens, clothing or textiles:

- Carefully remove any vomit or feces (poop) to minimize aerosols.
- Keep contaminated and uncontaminated clothes separate.
- Handle soiled linens and laundry as little as possible.
- Wash contaminated items in a pre-wash cycle. Then, use a regular wash cycle—using detergent—and dry separately from uncontaminated clothing at high temperature (greater than 170 degrees Fahrenheit).
- Make sure that all soiled linens, clothing or textiles are kept away from clean items.

For surfaces corrodible or damageable by bleach:

The Environmental Protection Agency recommends phenolic solutions (such as concentrated Lysol® or concentrated Pinesol®), mixed at two to four times the manufacturer's recommended concentration, as best for surfaces that could be damaged by bleach.

Source: Division of Environmental Health, N.C. Department of Environment and Natural Resources, Dec. 2008. Reviewed and adapted by Division of Public Health, N.C. Department of Health and Human Services, Oct. 2011.

For Additional Information

- NC DHHS: Personal Health Measures for the Prevention and Control of Norovirus (PDF, 61KB) - Updated October 2015

90

http://epi.publichealth.nc.gov/cd/norovirus/home.html